Beyond Food

The 5 Keys to Instant Health Without

Diets, Pills or Drastic Lifestyle Changes

———————————————

Marie Ann Mosher, CPT, AADP, CHHC

Beyond Food Publishing

Dedication

This book is dedicated to everyone who is overwhelmed by the idea of reclaiming health for themselves and their families. You CAN do it, and it's easier than you think!

Contents

How to Use This Book

I challenge you to read this book in its entirety. It is not necessary to believe or use everything in this book. Grab hold of the keys you think are useful and put them into action immediately! You will not have to implement all the action items and strategies in this book to transform the quality of your life. All the strategies and techniques have individual potential to change your life. When used together, however, they will produce amazing results that will stay with you for life.

I hope this will be a book you will read again and again. The purpose is to take your life to a whole new level. Please consider this book an indispensable tool with keys to upgrade your health for life.

Introduction

If you are like many Americans, you've spent a good portion of your adult life doing many unhealthy things. Not on purpose, of course. The demands of modern life – relentless careers, family obligations, social and volunteer commitments – all the things that keep us running from one task to the next virtually ensure that we put "making healthy choices" near the bottom of our to-do lists.

And why wouldn't we put it there? In a society where immediate results and streamlined efficiency are king and queen, taking the time to make healthy choices seems downright, well – inefficient! We are under the impression that exercising, eating well, and cooking simply take too much time. We drive around the corner to the store because it's quicker than walking. Once there, we buy boxes of processed and frozen foods we can throw in the microwave for the sake of convenience. We grab fast food, Chinese takeout, or order pizza delivery because it fills us up, it's cheap, and we don't have to clean up the kitchen.

Our work lives might be hectic, but they're also filled with conveniences that allow us to get our work done faster to make room for… more work! Telephones and computers mean we don't need to leave the office. We can e-mail instantly instead of going to the mailbox. We can text someone two floors down instead of going to see him in his office.

We might have a gym membership, but most of us don't use it. Most of us are too tired to even lace up the athletic shoes, much less get out the door. So most of us also do a lot of sitting at home, with our convenience and comfort foods on hand. We have our entertainment ready-made and delivered into our homes with the internet and the television. We shop online because what could be easier than just sitting on our sofas and finding what we want without even having to step outside our front door, much less walk from store to store in search of what we need? It's efficiency at its most efficient.

Not only does this way seem to be the most efficient course of action but even if we want to eat well, the principles of good nutrition are just too confusing to tackle. So, maybe we read a few articles, try the latest trick and fad. We get discouraged when it doesn't work or doesn't work for long, then go back to our comfortable, convenient habits.

Taking advantage of convenience seems to pay off for us in the moment. And yet in the end, we all pay a price for living this way.

You could make drastic lifestyle changes to avoid a potential tragedy, and if you make the right changes, it's incredibly effective. But it's not easy to do on our own, considering all the conflicting information out there – not to mention the considerable challenges involved with completely revamping a comfortable and familiar way of eating. In fact, a common refrain many of us sing when it comes to making healthy changes in our daily habits is, "I can't do that."

Well, of this you can be sure: if you consume the Standard American Diet on a regular basis, especially if coupled with a tendency to avoid physical activity as much as possible, a drastic lifestyle change awaits you anyway. It will come in the form of a heart attack, the discovery of diabetes, or cancer in one of its many forms. The body can handle being treated poorly for a long time, but only for just so long. Eventually, it will have no choice but to give in, and when it does, drastic lifestyle changes will be the result.

Though, they won't be changes you'll have taken charge of. The changes will have taken charge of you.

The good news is that you don't need to make a drastic change in your lifestyle to begin to make a profound difference in your health and your life starting today.

While no one eating plan works for everyone, there is one thing that's pretty much true across the board. Replace all that convenience in your life with authentic, rich, meaningful and joyful cooking, moving, working, and relating, and not only will you be healthier in your body, but your efficient existence will be transformed into a rewarding, vibrant life across the board.

Let me show you how.

Chapter One

Health Crisis

Unless you've been living under a rock for the past decade, you are well aware that we have a real crisis going on in our health care system. In fact, the odds are good you or someone you love has somehow been affected by this crisis.

Yet, when we use the term "health care," we typically aren't referring to health. We're talking about the economics of treating disease – the real difficulties involved with how much it costs to be covered by insurance, who can afford it, the quality of the coverage, and the high cost of co-pays and deductibles. We're speaking of the high cost of pharmaceutical drugs – who pays, who can afford them, and how many people need them. And we're also making reference to the high cost of the medical care itself – screenings and treatments and surgeries.

What's usually overlooked in the whole debate over the health CARE crisis is the primary reason why it's such a huge problem – a much more fundamental and dangerous HEALTH crisis. Comparatively speaking, we pay little attention to the underlying *causes* of these supposedly inevitable diseases and conditions that seem to eventually creep up on almost everyone – high blood pressure and cholesterol, diabetes, heart disease, strokes and cancer. We spend our time debating how to make all these procedures and medicines designed to treat their symptoms accessible and affordable, but we don't ask why so many people are looking to specialists, drugs, and surgical procedures to address their health concerns in the first place.

Why are we focusing on treatment to the exclusion of prevention?

The answer to that question is a complex formula of political special interests in the food and pharmaceutical industries, honest ignorance among the general public and even a good number of healthcare providers, and willful denial across the board in order to remain on the course of least resistance and maximum profit.

But the answer to the question, "What IS the cause of our nation's collective poor health?" is much simpler. The answer is food... or more accurately, our mass consumption of nutrient deficient food-like products manufactured in processing plants, combined with our lack of consumption of real whole foods grown on trees, nurtured in fields, and found in the ocean. The majority of what the government allows to pass for food in our grocery stores, restaurants and school cafeterias is easy to make and cheap to produce. What many of us end up eating most of the time are basically junk foods that do nothing to nourish us – and in fact, more often than not, do just the opposite. It's no coincidence that the alarming proliferation of conditions such as cancer, diabetes, obesity and heart disease has risen in direct proportion with the proliferation of the artificial and processed foods we eat. **Slowly but surely, the way we eat is killing us.**

The good news is that just as there is a clearly identifiable cause of our nation's collective health crisis, there's an equally identifiable solution to addressing it. If the cause of the problem is bad food, the solution to the problem is... good food! A new national consciousness that fosters the consumption of real, whole, nourishing foods would drastically change the nature of our discussion about how to solve the health care crisis.

Just imagine:

What if you only went to see your doctor for routine physicals and screenings, or when you break a bone or suffer some kind of unavoidable (and hopefully rare) injury?

What if when it comes to cancer, instead of a "race for the cure," we began a "push for prevention?"

What if you could not only easily find your way to the weight that's comfortable for you, but you could also practically ensure you wouldn't have a heart attack, end up with cancer, raise your blood pressure, suffer from diabetes, deal with poor digestion, or find yourself afflicted with any of the self-imposed conditions that plague our nation and comprise the majority of our country's mortality rate?

What if you could just expect to live a long, healthy, happy life that ends naturally and peacefully when it's supposed to?

You can. Most people can. Just eat real food!

Real, nourishing, delicious whole foods have been proven to build bodies that thrive, and minds that are sharp.

Research and experience proves that they prevent cancer, heart disease, and diabetes. They can even, in some cases, make such conditions go away! They prevent and reverse acid reflux, attention deficit disorder, high cholesterol, and high blood pressure. Food is the answer to prevention. It's the miracle cure. It's the solution that's been right under our noses all along.

And before you begin to think that you might have done too much damage already by your food choices in the past, it's never too late to begin making healthy choices that matter. The body is remarkably adaptable, and its natural inclination is to be healthy. So, when we support this inclination with healthy habits and behaviors, we see a difference, and we see it quickly.

Food isn't the only component of health, of course. But it's the first one. Get that right, and the others will follow. This is an exciting time to be alive. There is a small but growing movement that understands the role real food plays in our health. Why don't you join us? You can be a pioneer on the road to genuine HEALTH reform, making a difference first in your own life, then in your family, community, and world. And it starts by simply choosing to eat real food!

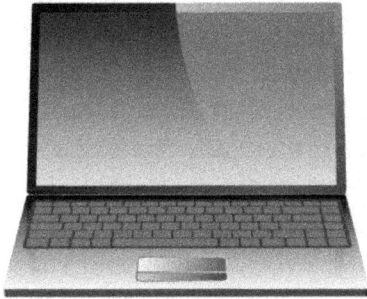

Key #1

Awareness !

Are you eating junk or are you eating REAL food? Start first by keeping a journal. Intention and awareness is everything. Keeping track of what you eat and how you feel will give you invaluable data and insight into your patterns and reasons for why you do the things you do. Did you eat that pint of ice cream because you were hungry? Thirsty? Lonely? It can be a powerful exercise to explore your motivations in this way.

Writing down your intentions is even more powerful – if you put something you plan to do in writing, you are simply more likely to do it.

It also helps immensely to track how foods make us feel after we eat them. After you ate that pint of ice cream, for instance, how did your body respond? Were you more alert? Hyper? Lethargic? Bloated? Did you feel restless, unsatisfied, and even hungrier? How different do you feel after eating a salad, a bowl of oatmeal, or a plate of scrambled eggs? Do you feel grounded and at peace? Light and refreshed? Are you hungry and wanting something more?

Over time, recording the way your body responds to food will help you see patterns and learn what works and doesn't work for you. It will also help you understand how food works on a much deeper level in affecting your entire well being, far beyond the choices you make to satisfy your taste buds and fleeting emotions in that moment.

Use a writing system that works for you – a simple notebook will do. Even better use a word processing program or a Smartphone application. Send emails or texts to yourself. Whatever form of written expression works best for you, do it.

The point is to keep a record – first of the foods you eat, and then of the exercise you undertake, the joys and stresses you encounter at work, the spiritual practices you adopt, the state of your relationships, etc. Write a record of how things are, and also take the time to write how you'd like things to be.

Here's an example of how one person's journal entry might look on a given day:

Today, I drank more water than usual, ate a big salad at lunch and skipped the bread, and had strawberries instead of cookies after dinner. I felt better after eating the fruit than I usually do after eating cookies, which always make me want to eat more. I plan to give up my coffee tomorrow. I find I reach for that coffee in the mornings after the staff meeting at 9:30 and load it with cream and sugar, so when the urge hits for that cup of coffee, I'm going to have some water and take a quick five minute walk instead. Jason had a hard day at work yesterday, so it felt good to spend a little time with him tonight just letting him talk. And Jessica was having trouble with her homework. I'd gotten angry with her for not doing it, but after a few deep breaths, I was able to step back and give her a hand. All in all, I'm happy with today's progress, and I look forward to tomorrow.

This is just a quick narrative of how the day went and the hopes for how it will go tomorrow. Do this sort of thing in whatever style works for you, and you'll be amazed at what you learn about yourself, and how much you will grow.

Chapter Two

Eating Well
Principles that Apply to All of Us

"Eat food. Not too much. Mostly plants."

For all the millions of pages written about eating well, these seven words sum it up best. This quote from Michael Pollan, the author of *The Omnivore's Dilemma*, captures the essence of what we need to know to enjoy a long, healthy life.

"Eat food." By this, he means REAL food. The kind of food that comes from nature, that grows in the ground or on trees or on the ocean floor. Food that comes from animals who are treated well and not poisoned with chemicals or whose products come to us tainted by how they are raised, slaughtered, and processed. This is the kind of food that will go bad if you don't eat it within a few days, because it's not been fortified with artificial preservatives intended to ensure a long shelf life (and as few nutrients as possible).

Remember this helpful adage: the longer the shelf life of a food you eat, the shorter YOUR shelf life will be. If you can't pronounce the ingredients on a food label without a chemistry degree, then it is NOT healthy!

"Not too much." The majority of us simply eat too much food. The amount of food (and calories) presented on your average restaurant plate in America is astounding. Portion control, no matter what any diet plan says, is important. It's not about deprivation or starving yourself, though. It's about eating the right amount – no more, no less.

"Mostly plants." Certainly, some people find nourishment, comfort, and strength from animal products like meat, fish, and dairy. But most of us eat far more of these kinds of foods than our bodies can possibly process and properly digest. And many of us cannot only live without them, but we thrive when we replace them with plant-based foods. When we eat high nutrient foods, we find that not only are our bellies full and satisfied, but we feel their effects throughout our bodies – and beyond.

So, how can we begin to put Pollan's simple little philosophy into practice? Here are the principles that, generally speaking, apply to all of us.

Start with greens

Greens, greens, and lots of them! Greens are the most nutrient dense foods on the planet. The darker, the better. Eating salads helps ensure you get a lot of your greens raw. When cooking, steam them briefly – or you can even bake them on a low heat in the oven for a crispy chip-like texture.

Add a wide variety of vegetables to your meals.

There are so many options in the produce department, so here's a chance to experiment with new flavors. Eggplants, squash, zucchini, carrots, sweet potatoes, onions, mushrooms, cucumbers, radishes… the list goes on and on. If you are unaccustomed to eating vegetables, it might take a little while to get your palate adjusted to their tastes and textures. But the key to getting all the various vitamins and nutrients available is color. A variety of colors every day will ensure a good mix of different nutrients to fuel your body exceptionally well.

Make sure your body is hydrated.

This means hydrated with water, not DEhydrated by coffee, soda, beer, or other drinks. Conventional wisdom says 64 ounces a day is an ideal amount. But you need to let your body dictate how much water consumption is optimal for you.

Lots of greens, lots of vegetables, and adequate water – are the most universally applicable rules. The following are generally applicable:

Fruits: Most of us should eat a serving or two of fruit a day. Foods like berries provide a huge dose of antioxidants. Apples are a good source of fiber, bananas give us potassium, avocados have healthy fats… every fruit has several benefits, in fact. A word of caution, however, for people with diabetes or other blood sugar issues: Most fruits do contain fructose, and this can be problematic in the diets of some people. Though the sugar is natural, sugar is sugar. It can lead to weight gain or other more serious complications, so leaning more toward low fructose fruits are your best bet. And moderation is key.

Whole grains: Whole grains are the unprocessed kind, not the highly refined and "enriched" products we see in the bags of white sandwich bread and boxes of "instant" white rice on the supermarket shelves. "Refined" and "enriched" sound like such positive words, but don't be fooled. Refined grain has been stripped of its raw nutrients and does little more than spike your blood sugar through its empty calories. It tends to be "white" food, or sometimes colored with an artificial ingredient to cover up its "whiteness," as in the case with many so-called "wheat" breads.

A good rule of thumb is to avoid foods such as white rice, white breads, pastas and even possibly white potatoes. Try red or sweet potatoes for a change, brown rice instead of white, and be adventurous with other grains as well – it's not hard to find tasty recipes that call for quinoa, millet, and barley. Truly whole grain breads have very few ingredients besides the grains themselves. You can even find live sprouted grain breads that don't have flour, which are excellent sources of protein and fiber.

Beans and legumes: These nutrient powerhouses are tremendously high in protein and fiber. If you aren't used to eating them, you may experience a bit of digestive discomfort at first. But as your overall diet improves over time, that tends to ease up. There are endless varieties of soups, casseroles, dips and Mexican dishes you can prepare starting with beans.

Nuts and Seeds: Avoid the roasted, salted, and oiled kinds. And of course, if you're allergic, avoid them in all forms. But for the rest of us, raw nuts and seeds, as well as nut and seed butters, are excellent sources of protein and nutrients, and they also aid in the absorption of nutrients from greens in smoothies and salads.

Nuts in particular are high in calories and should be enjoyed in moderation – a handful is an adequate serving for most of us.

A diet of greens, vegetables, fruits, whole grains, beans, legumes, nuts and seeds – along with adequate water intake – is a fantastic foundation for our overall eating plan. With very few exceptions, a diet consisting of just these foods can get our weight quickly under control, prevent all our modern lifestyle diseases, and even reverse them in people who already have them. Many people – former President Bill Clinton is perhaps the most famous example – stick to this way of eating and have no desire or need to consume anything else, while protecting themselves from cancer, heart attacks, diabetes, and a whole host of other health concerns.

But, while consuming more of these foods is a health benefit to almost everyone, eating only these foods doesn't work for everyone. In the next chapter, we'll have some suggestions for figuring out how to develop an individualized eating plan that works specifically for YOU.

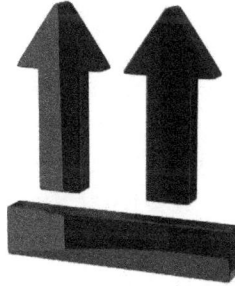

Key #2

Upgrade your Foods !

If there were only one thing you could do for your health to make a truly noticeable difference right away, and a lasting difference for the rest of your life, I'd recommend you learn how to make and enjoy a daily green smoothie – or two. A favorite of third graders who also enjoy cakes that look like soil with gummy worms emerging through the surface, green smoothies tend, on first sight, not to appeal to adults with more seemingly refined tastes.

That's because they're green, and for some reason, too many of us adults have lost our sense of adventure. Once an adult closes his eyes and tastes a green smoothie, though, it's a different story. When blended properly, it's a delightfully refreshing treat that transcends the color in the glass. And when you realize all the health benefits of drinking green smoothies, you won't want to live without them.

Why Greens?

We've all enjoyed fruit smoothies as a quick breakfast or a snack. You'll find plenty of juice bars and other shops that sell smoothies these days as a healthier alternative to the other fast food options out there. And that's a good thing. Fruit is important for our bodies, so smoothies provide an awesome source of fiber and essential nutrients. Some, like berries, are also an excellent source of antioxidants, which help fight infection and disease. Most of us don't get enough fruit in our daily diets, and smoothies are a great way to add them.

But the problem with most smoothies sold in retail outlets is what they add – extra sugar and dairy. And very few of them contain the most nutrient dense foods on the planet: leafy green vegetables.

Foods like spinach, kale, collards, swiss chard, bok choy, watercress, parsley, mustard greens, turnip greens – these are the foods with the most nutrients in the purest form, with the fewest amount of calories per serving. Want to lose weight? Eat your greens!

As we know, Americans eat fewer leafy green vegetables than any other food. We need them the most, but eat them the least, and our waistlines are proof.

You might be thinking, "Okay, I'll eat more greens. But put them in a smoothie? That's disgusting!" Actually, it's a surprisingly easy and delicious way to eat them – especially if you don't like them, or haven't gotten your taste buds accustomed to them yet. The taste is hardly noticeable when blended with fruits, so it's not as off-putting in your glass as it might seem at first in the blender.

Speaking of the blender…

Why Blend It?

There are several reasons why blending is not only a convenient way to get your greens, but also a superior way:

1.   **Quantity**: To get the most out of eating leafy greens, you need to eat a LOT of them. This is actually a time consuming task, and unless you love greens more than any other food in the world and plan to eat several large salads a day, you aren't likely to eat them in the quantities that will deliver serious health benefits.

You may find that you are able to consume up to three times as many greens in a smoothie as you are in a salad or steamed dish.

2.   **Taste**: Thanks to our modern processed diet, many of us have a hard time appreciating the flavors of greens. Some of us love them, but for the many more who don't, hiding greens in a smoothie is the perfect way to eat them without tasting them.

3.   **Benefits of Raw**: There is a lot of evidence pointing to the benefits of eating raw foods. Most plants, when cooked, tend to lose their nutrients and digestive enzymes to varying degrees, depending on the temperature at which they are cooked, the method, etc. Since the greens in your smoothie are always raw, you get the benefit of all the nutrients in their purest whole food state.

4.   **Digestion**: Greens are called roughage for a reason; they can be pretty rough on our intestinal tracts. And when we chew, we don't always get all the benefits of the food.

According to Dr. Joel Fuhrman, longtime advocate of achieving nutritional excellence through the consumption of a plant-based diet: "When we simply chew a salad, about 70 to 90 percent of the [plant] cells are not broken open. As a result, most of the valuable nutrients contained within those cells never enter our bloodstream." He considers what he calls a "blended salad" a "powerful and delicious way to maximize your intake of nutrients."

Since the food in a smoothie has already been mostly pulverized from going through the blender, your body will digest the food much more easily, and assimilate the nutrients much faster. Once the nutrients are in your system, you often feel the difference in terms of energy and well being immediately.

Green Smoothie Recipes

You can go ahead and buy a green smoothie recipe book if you like. But green smoothies are the easiest meals in the world to make. Basically, you just throw everything in a blender and press the button. Most of us have a blender. (If you've only ever used yours for making frozen cocktails, it's just as easy to make a smoothie – and certainly much more healthy!) All you need are a few taste preferences – and a little common sense. So here is the most basic recipe for maximum ease, powerful nutrition, and fantastic taste.

The Basic Three Minute Green Smoothie

You'll need:

•   **A blender.** The higher powered, the better. But really, any blender that works will do the trick. Don't delay simply because you don't have a Vitamix on your kitchen counter!

•   **Up to eight cups of loose, leafy green vegetables.** The amount is purely based on what you want to achieve. If you want to ease into the smoothies and are a bit apprehensive about the taste of them in a blended drink, a handful of spinach is a great place to start. If you want to be amazed by the jolt of energy and clarity you'll feel after drinking one, you'll want to fill your blender (loosely!) to the top with one or more of the variety of greens listed earlier in this chapter.

34

- **One or two ripe bananas**
- **A 12 or 16 oz bag of frozen fruit** – just be sure there is NOTHING added to the bag besides pure fruit
- **3 cups of pure water** (more or less to taste)

The key to the smoothie is blending it well. While we all have our preferences, a super chunky smoothie really doesn't appeal to too many people.

1. Start by filling your blender with the greens, then add the water and blend thoroughly. If you've filled the blender to the top with the greens, the volume should come down about halfway after being blended.
2. Peel and add the bananas. You may want to start with one and see how full your blender becomes. But if the bananas are small, be sure to add the second for the creamy consistency and natural sweetness necessary to counter the taste of any greens. After a while, you may be able to reduce the number of bananas to make room for more greens.
3. Add your bag of fruit. Because the fruit is frozen, the nutrients are just as powerful, if not more so, than in fresh fruit. The convenience of a frozen bag of fruit can't be denied – no peeling, no washing, and no mess. And the frozen factor means you don't have to add ice to make the smoothie cold.

The first few times you do this, you may find you have to experiment a bit with the amounts of water and greens that feel right to you. So be patient, and give yourself a bit of time to figure it out.

Adding Other Ingredients

This is the basic, simple, straightforward, nutrient powerhouse smoothie. While you don't need to add other ingredients, you might want to, for the benefit of taste or nutrition. If you're looking for more flavor, try an all-natural fruit juice. Orange or apple juice would be simple, but there are lots of exotic options out there too, such as mango, pineapple, or pomegranate. Just stay away from anything that contains added sugar, syrup, or preservatives. Stick with a 100% natural juice.

If you want a more creamy consistency, you might try soy, coconut, hemp or almond milk. Some people prefer yogurt or cow's milk. Be aware that many people are intolerant of cow dairy products and don't even know it, so using such ingredients might negate the benefits of the whole foods in your smoothie. Also keep in mind that adding any liquid besides water will add calories – there is no way around that one.

If you want to add layers of nutrition, you can certainly add other fresh fruits and vegetables – any of them will work. Perhaps you'd like the kick of a jalapeno pepper in yours, or one of your kids can't stand the taste of carrots but you want her to benefit from their nutritional value. These additions do require the power of a top-notch blender. You can use frozen vegetables as well – you just need to let the vegetables thaw a bit before subjecting your blender to them. Frozen vegetables aren't completely raw… they are very quickly blanched before freezing, so while they don't lose much in the way of nutrients, they aren't exactly as powerful as raw.

And some people swear by adding a bit of healthy fat to their smoothies – some coconut oil, almond butter, or avocado, for instance. Fats do help aid in the absorption of nutrients. This can also be achieved by eating a small handful of nuts along with your smoothie.

One other note: switch up your greens every few days. If you blended nothing but kale for a week, for instance, you might bring on an alkaloid build up in your system, which isn't optimal for your health. Using different greens throughout the week will prevent that from happening.

The possibilities and combinations are endless if you really want to be adventurous. There are lots of books on the market and resources on the web to help you sort through the options. Have fun checking them all out!

When and How To Enjoy

Like many modern day Americans, you may feel like you don't have time for breakfast. Well, now you do, and research suggests that eating plants first thing in the morning is an extremely healthy way to start your day. Three minutes are all it takes to whip up this recipe if you want it fresh. You can prepare it the night before and have it ready if you or your family isn't willing to endure the early morning noise. If you've made a whole pitcher, you might also try filling a portable shaker bottle so you can enjoy one at work before lunch, for lunch, or as a snack. Just store it in a refrigerator, and leave enough room in the bottle to be able to shake the contents, as they will settle and thicken over the course of a few hours.

Marie's TIP

Take a few minutes in the grocery store to pick up these ingredients, set aside a little time in your kitchen to play with your blender, and enjoy the amazingly healthy – and delicious – results!

Chapter Three

You Are Unique

Now that we know the basic foods everyone should eat, how do we figure out the rest? If we each have a different body that needs different foods in different amounts, how can we know exactly what to do?

Well, one thing NOT to do is to buy just any book on healthful eating and follow it religiously. Have you ever noticed how many diet and healthy eating books are on the shelves of your local bookstore? It's overwhelming, and new books, studies, and programs are developed all the time. Each one claims to have the cure to losing weight / staying young / building muscle / gaining energy in its pages. Give up carbs, restrict calories, eat low fat, eat high fat, cut out sugar, eat at certain times, eat this but not that, go vegan, go raw, load up on protein. You can eat for your blood type, rate every food you eat on the glycemic index, try the Atkins plan, cure your belly fat, or eat to address hormonal imbalances.

Every theory is backed up by some kind of empirical evidence, years of research and trials and proof that they work.

The truth is, if any one of these plans had THE answer to achieving optimum health for everyone, it would be the ONLY plan.

All these books have made it on the shelves of the bookstores for two reasons. One, because each one of these plans HAS worked for SOMEONE. And two, because the rest of us are looking for the plan that will work for US.

You can certainly read all those books, and the odds are good one of them will provide the basic elements of an eating style you can live with - and maybe even thrive with - for the rest of your life. But how will you know which diet is right for you?

To start with, you won't. It will take time, patience, and a willingness to experiment with foods you love while determining which ones also love you back. Also remember – don't eat foods that you are allergic to or intolerant of. And if something makes you feel bad, don't eat it! Keep journaling and working this out for yourself, and in time, you'll have written your own diet book – the one that applies just to you.

As noted in the previous chapter, a few basics apply. Whole foods, mostly plants, eaten in great abundance, are the best weapons to prevent and even reverse disease as well as upgrade the quality of your life.

Beyond that, it's up to each of us to figure out what works in other food groups. Some people can figure this out on their own, but it requires patience and experimentation. Just as there are several ways of eating, there are several ways of beginning to determine the best way of eating for you:

1.	Crowding out. Instead of eliminating things from your diet, make a conscious effort to incorporate more good things. If you don't usually eat salads, you could add one to your lunch every day. Try the green smoothies, and resolve to drink at least one serving a day. Add in a handful of carrots, change from salted mixed nuts to raw almonds and walnuts, eat an apple in the afternoons, drink an extra glass of water a day – these are just a few examples of ways you can add healthy habits into your routine. Add enough of them in, and you'll have no choice but to crowd out the less healthy choices.

2.	Gradually eliminate things from your diet based on bad habits you want to conquer or ailments from which you are suffering. For instance, if you feel sluggish, you might want to try eliminating dairy from your diet for a week.

If you haven't been eating breakfast and want to figure out what will best get your motor going in the mornings, spend a week trying different foods for breakfast, and making notes about the effects they have on your energy, digestion, and sense of mental clarity.

Some people thrive on green smoothies, others prefer the grounding properties of a warm bowl of rolled oats with fruit. Still others find the protein in fresh eggs to be an essential staple in a healthy morning breakfast.

3.   Do a whole foods detox, then experiment by adding things back in. If you have the discipline and determination to spend at least five days detoxing your body with a whole foods, plant-based, smoothie and/or juice detox, your body will be more aware of how other foods affect it. Be sure to add other foods in one at a time, so you know what food is having what kind of effect on you. Reintroduce dairy one week, meat the next. You may even find after detoxing that you no longer have a taste for certain foods you used to crave.

No matter what style of eating works for you, the main premise is that a high nutrient diet is critical.

Try this one day sample menu intended to get flavorful, super nutrient dense foods into your diet. Again, you might not find that you enjoy all these foods, or your body might not tolerate them. But until you try and experiment, you won't know.

• *Breakfast:* Large green smoothie, raw almond butter with all natural fruit jam on sprouted grain toast, herbal tea

• *Lunch:* Small green smoothie or pure vegetable juice, huge salad with your favorite veggies, fruits, nuts and greens, balsamic vinaigrette dressing, one slice of pizza - mushrooms and peppers with goat cheese on whole grain crust or grain free crust

• *Snack:* Handful of walnuts with raisins

• *Dinner:* Mexican vegetable and bean soup flavored with cilantro, whole grain tortillas with salsa and black beans

• *Dessert:* strawberry-chocolate smoothie – recipe below:

¼ cup coconut milk, ¼ cup pure water, 5 dates, pitted and soaked in the water, ¼ avocado, 1 cup of fresh spinach, 1 tablespoon of raw cacao, ¼ cup frozen strawberries

Pour the milk and water into the blender with the dates, avocado, and cacao on top. Blend. Add the spinach and strawberries and blend until completely smooth. Serves 1-2.

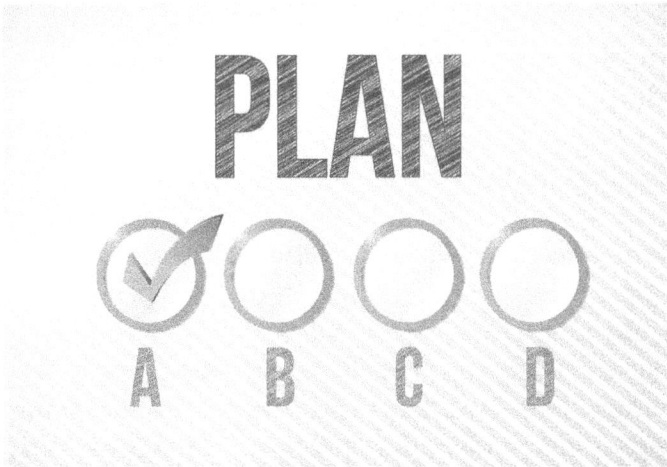

Key #3

Prepare For Success !

Have you convinced yourself that you are too busy to eat well? No time for breakfast (before you learned about the smoothies!) or no time for lunch? Maybe some days your body goes into "starvation mode" by lunchtime, and you don't want to eat a thing. On other days, you might be ravenously hungry by noon, and all you want are a burger and some fries. Odds are good your office is filled with snacks that can sabotage the best intentions: cookies and chips, vending machines with processed foods, sodas and candy. Sound at all familiar?

Managing hunger and nutrition during the workday seems daunting at first, but it simply requires a little planning ahead of time. Knowing how busy you are, these are some of the best and most convenient foods to keep handy at your workplace for those instances when it seems all forces in the world are conspiring against your doing what's best for you. Head to the store and purchase these according to your tastes and storage options in your office. And keep them out of reach of your coworkers and visitors for now. Remember, you have to be healthy first!

1.   **Nuts and Seeds**. These are the best and most convenient all natural snacks you can keep around. Unlike fruits and vegetables, they keep for some time. You can buy them in bulk and not worry about running to the store every few days to replenish them. Stock up on the raw, unsalted varieties you like. Almonds and walnuts have tremendous health benefits, as do sunflower and sesame seeds.

If you are watching your weight, stick to just a handful a day, as the natural fats, although healthy, can work against a plan to lose weight. Slivered almonds might be preferable to the whole kind in this instance. Quite often I mix a handful of sprouted nuts and seeds with raisins, which makes for a very satisfying and healthy protein rich snack with a variety of tastes in a small portion.

2.   **Veggie trays and dips**. Vegetables actually make fantastic snacks, even more so when paired with a tasty dip. Carrots, celery, cucumbers and broccoli might be a bit challenging to get into your blender, but you can find them conveniently cut and packaged in the produce section of almost any grocery store. They also tend to be paired in those packages with a dip that is based in a processed, high fat ranch dressing, which isn't exactly optimal for health. So, I recommend you find a nice hummus dip to complement this snack. Made from garbanzo beans, it's a delicious way to spice up the vegetables that might be lacking the flavors your taste buds are used to. They make all kinds of hummus these days, too – with garlic, pine nuts, lemon, roasted peppers, you name it.

You can find other healthy dips if hummus isn't your thing or you want to mix things up – there are some great bean dips (not the refried kind!), delicious guacamole and all natural salsas ranging from mild to super hot. If you're inclined, of course you could make all these dips yourself. But if you're pressed for time and want the "convenience" factor, you can find all these foods prepared and packaged without preservatives or artificial ingredients. Read the ingredient labels and purchase something that clearly shows only whole foods in the list.

3.   **Peanut Butter and Jelly**. What could be more nostalgic than to put a nice peanut butter and jelly sandwich in your lunch box? This is a much healthier – and in my opinion, tastier – version than the Wonder Bread – Jiffy – Smuckers combination most of us remember from childhood. It's easy to prepare, wrap, and take with you every day as a filling, healthy, protein filled lunch or snack. Live sprouted grain breads, like Ezekiel or Whole Food's brand, are becoming more and more popular. If you can't find it right away, look for the loaves in your grocer's freezer. It's comprised of live sprouted grains, not enriched wheat flour that's been stripped of its nutrients. These breads are a super source of protein, made from freshly sprouted organically grown grains and legumes. The breads are naturally rich in (as opposed to artificially fortified with) protein, vitamins, minerals and fiber with no added fat.

If you simply can't find it, speak to the store manager about stocking it, and head to the bakery – not the factory processed bread aisle – to find a truly whole grain bread. Spread a couple of slices with some all natural peanut or preferably almond butter (no sugar added, just nuts) and an all-natural fruit spread – again, with NO SUGAR ADDED.

4.   **Five apples and five bananas.** These traditional, common fruits are easy to bring, eat, and dispose of. No need for a knife to peel. Take your time and pick out the best looking apples you can find – and if you like and don't mind peeling, find some other fruits, too.

Set up a bowl on your desk to store them. The attractive arrangement will also brighten your mood the way a fresh bouquet of flowers or a sturdy plant would.

5.   **Whole food bars.** There have been lots of energy and meal replacement bars on the market for decades now. The problem with most of them is that they are highly processed and laden with sugar and high fructose corn syrup. They won't help your health goals any more than a Snickers bar would.

Brands such as Larabar, Pure Bar, and Amazing Greens (to name a few) have developed the technology to produce whole food bars without any of those artificial or sugary ingredients. Lots of these bars come in chocolate varieties, flavored with nutrient rich cacao and sweetened with dried fruit. Again, read labels religiously.

And if you want to make your own, here's a ridiculously simple recipe for raw vegan brownies that will take as long to make as it does for you to get from the power bar section in your grocery store, through the checkout, and into your car!

1 cup of pitted mejool dates
1 cup of walnuts
¼ cup of cacao powder

Blend all of the above in a blender or food processor and press into a small baking dish. Refrigerate or freeze. Makes nine small but very filling brownies.

Another sweet treat? Take the above ingredients and after blending, instead of pressing into a pan, crumble and sprinkle over fresh raspberries. Decadently healthy!

6.   **All natural chips and crackers.**
Sometimes, we do crave a little salt and a little crunch. If you can handle eating them in moderation, look in the snack section for products that are few in ingredients, and whose ingredients begin with whole grains. There are certain crackers, tortilla and rice chips on the market that fit the bill and also pair nicely with the aforementioned salsas and hummus dips.

Better yet, try to make some crunchy, salty things on your own, like kale chips! Just remove the leaves from the stems, coat them with a little grapeseed oil, bake for five to ten minutes at 350 degrees, then sprinkle with some sea salt as soon as you remove them. Delicious!

Try to make an effort to drink your smoothies and eat these snacks before you indulge in any other foods around the office, especially when special occasions pop up to sabotage your efforts to eat better.

Don't skip the foods on holidays or other treats you might like if you want them. But you may just find that with a smoothie or two, a handful of carrots, and that spectacular peanut butter and jelly sandwich in your system, those other foods don't appeal to you quite the way they did before. Amazing what real food can do!

Sneaky Calories!

Almost all Americans have a drinking problem. Alcohol addictions notwithstanding, I'm mostly talking about our consumption of drinks laden with caffeine, sugar, and artificial sweeteners. Many studies actually point to the fact that it's our drinking habits more than our eating habits that pack on the calories and the pounds.

Americans are notorious for walking around the office with the ubiquitous cup of coffee in the mornings, often with cream and sugar. And many follow in the afternoons with soda to keep going – high test or the diet kind, either kind of soft drink is again filled with additives, preservatives, high fructose corn syrup or artificial sweeteners proven to cause cancer in rats and suspected to do the same in humans.

As bad as the sugar, cream, and aspartame can be, the caffeine itself is addictive and suspected of contributing to a whole host of health concerns.

Of course, there are studies that also point to some possible health benefits of caffeine and coffee, so the data really is inconclusive. But any potential benefits of caffeine come from moderate consumption, not addiction.

In any case, virtually every American walks through his or her day in a state of dehydration. We simply don't drink enough of the one and only drink Mother Nature provides us completely free of charge: water.

The standard recommendation of eight 8 ounce glasses a day doesn't exactly apply to everyone; we all have varying levels of need for water, and it takes a while to figure out what works for each of us.

If you take the time to work through how and what you drink during the day, you'll probably be surprised by the difference you'll feel in no time.

1.   **Water**. Add one full glass of water to your day, preferably early in the morning. In fact, if you are able to consume 16 ounces in the morning on an empty stomach, you'll get the incomparable benefit of a daily early morning detox. And you'll notice a difference as early as day one!

Perhaps you can bring a big bottle to sit on your desk and sip it throughout the day, or find another means of H2O delivery that works for you. But if you aren't drinking enough, don't start out trying to drink a gallon at once. It won't work. Try one glass a day, and see how it feels to you.

2.   **Coffee and Tea**. If you are a coffee addict, or even if you stick to one or two cups a day, try a cup of tea this morning. Flavor it however you like – preferably naturally! – but experiment with something other than just coffee beans: chai tea, green tea, white tea, or any of the dozens of herbal teas on the market.
        Many kinds of teas are much lower in caffeine and high in antioxidants. Some are also known to calm the nerves, which is often the exact opposite of the effect that coffee has.

3.   **Soda**. There are different reasons why people drink soda. It would be a good idea for you to take some time to examine what your reasons are. It might be that it's a convenient option in a nearby vending machine. If that's the case, again it goes back to planning ahead to make provisions for yourself.

If it's the "fizz factor," there are lots of carbonated drinks that can fit the bill, without all the unhealthy side effects. Try simple sparkling mineral water, or a version flavored with lemon, lime, or raspberries. (All natural, of course! No sugar, syrup, or aspartame!)

If you really want a sweet taste, try this half and half recipe: fill your glass halfway with sparkling water, and halfway with your favorite all natural fruit juice.

There is also a soda on the market (not yet widely available) that effectively uses Stevia, an all-natural plant sweetener, to produce a remarkably sweet soda that you might enjoy if you're just not ready to kick the habit. If you drink soda, try drinking one of these alternatives in the afternoon at a time when you'd ordinarily grab that Coke or diet Pepsi. And if you like, experiment with all the options until you find the one that works the best for you.

Notice this plan doesn't call for you to give up your coffee, soda, or sweet tea. Just add these three drinks to your day – one glass of water, one cup of tea, and one sparkling drink. Give it some time to see how these might become new habits you'll want to keep. And maybe after a while, you'll even find you won't want to hang on to the old ones.

Chapter Four

Lifestyle Balance

The food we eat is foundational. It really can change everything – especially the way we feel, both physically and mentally. Of course, these good feelings can also lead to many other areas of improvement in our lives. And they often do. Recent studies have even shown that longevity might actually have more to do with these other areas in our lives than with the food we eat.

It all goes together. If you start eating well, you give yourself the best possible foundation for a well-functioning machine (your body) that can handle the particulars of all the other truly more important aspects of your life.

These are strange times we live in. On the one hand, we are living on average almost twice as long as our ancestors lived a hundred years ago. Twice as long! That's an amazing leap in life expectancy.

We certainly do owe a lot of that to science and modern medicine, to the eradication of many diseases, and to surgical procedures and pharmaceuticals that allow us to confront mortal dangers in ways unthinkable throughout most of human history.

And yet, most of us spend the last few years of our longer lives battling diseases that we brought on ourselves - diseases that were unheard of in generations past. Heart disease is the number one killer, followed closely by cancer and strokes come in at number three. We blindly accept these conditions as a normal part of growing older, because "we're all going to die from something."

I'm not so sure this is "living" longer. It's existing, but is it truly living? And death from "natural causes" is a very rare cause of death these days indeed.

It's no surprise, though, that we resign ourselves to that sort of death. It's a logical end to the kind of lives so many of us lead - more of an 'existence' for the sake of surviving, not thriving.

We run from one moment to the next, satisfying needs and wants based on the premise of immediate gratification, without taking much time to look at the whole picture in our lives.

We rush out the door to work in the morning, plow through the stresses of the tasks before us in fear of losing our jobs because we have bills to pay, not because the work has any deeper meaning for us.

We grab the food that's most convenient and tastes good to our dulled taste buds, not the foods our bodies need to thrive. We rarely sit down to eat, and when we do, we're often alone, in front of the television or computer, mindless images and entertainment taking up valuable space in our brains.

We sit far more often than we stand, drive when we could walk, take elevators when the stairs are right there. We spend more time texting than talking, taking our spouses for granted and forgetting to participate in our children's growth to adulthood.

How many of us truly take the time to meditate, to think, to pray, to be?

We are each given one precious life. And if we're really going to live it, we need to have a holistic approach to it. Health and happiness don't just happen. We must look at all aspects of our lives.

Eating well is critically important, but it alone cannot fill our souls.

"Primary Food" is a term coined by Joshua Rosenthal, founder of the groundbreaking Institute for Integrative Nutrition. Primary Foods encompass those areas of our lives that make us complete people and that must be filled in healthy ways, lest we use the wrong things to somehow try and fill the void. These key areas of our lives are spirituality, relationships, work and movement.

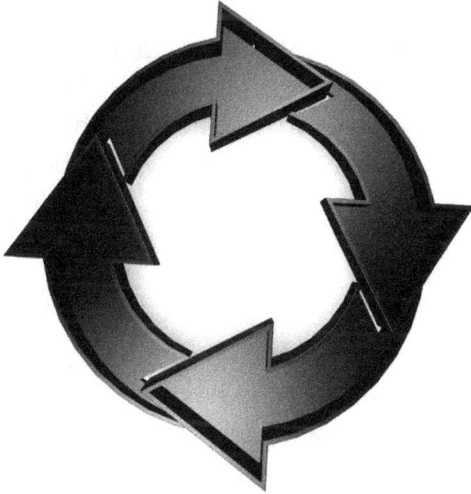

Key #4

Balance Your Circle of Life

Spirituality

Human civilizations throughout history have sought to make sense of our existence and find ultimate meaning. Across cultures, there has almost universally been an understanding of a higher power, a force greater than ourselves - and the need exists to connect with this force in order to reach our potential as humans. There is a deep and profound need for us to nourish a rich spiritual life.

Unfortunately, the pace of the modern world conspires to keep us from doing this at almost every turn.

Spirituality means different things to different people. It may mean a specific prayer life, attendance at church, spending quiet time alone on one's porch, reconnecting with nature on a hike through the woods, reflecting on choices made or that need to be made, being quiet and meditating, reading books about inspirational people who have made a difference in the world, getting lost in sacred music, yoga or a combination of practices... the list is endless.

If you are struggling with your own spiritual journey, it might take some time to figure out what is right for you. To start, just turn off the noise in your life - the television, the computer, the music, the mundane tasks in your job, the grumpy neighbors, all of it. Find a quiet place, and just focus on being in the moment - even if it's only for a few moments.

This is a great place to start, allowing yourself to be open to listening to another still voice that will feed your soul with what's good for you, instead of the external noise that will distract you from it. Give it time and be open to the promptings of the Spirit, and you'll begin to find the books and the people who can support you on your spiritual journey to figure out what the next steps are for you.

Relationships

Relationships are so sadly fractured in our society, and frequently misunderstood. It's been said that in our world today, we often love things and use people, when it should be the other way around. Love is unconditional, deep, sometimes challenging, rooted in kindness but also truth. It is perhaps the most important ingredient to a happy life.

But we suffer from a poverty of love in our world. Too many children grow up with inattentive parents, who more often than not are single or temporarily partnered with someone who isn't the other parent of those children - because that previous relationship was disposable.

Elderly people are with increasing frequency abandoned to nursing homes because their children are too busy to care for them. We tend to move too often, every few years, which ensures that the establishment of neighborhood communities and long lasting friendships cannot be possible.

None of this is intended to lay blame, but there's a lot of sadness in our world today when it comes to relationships.

And this is sad, but are love and relationships really connected to our health? Well, we can see it right at the start of our lives. Babies who are not held and loved at birth will die, and those who get very little of it often grow up seriously mal-adjusted. Research shows that good, strong relationships simply keep us healthy. They keep stress at bay and thus prevent illnesses brought on by stress.

People who have the benefit of loving spouses or partners, who are close to their children and parents, who cultivate a meaningful network of friends and family - these things are even more important than eating your recommended requirement of greens every day.

We could eat all the healthiest foods in the world, but if we don't have meaningful relationships in our lives, then what are we really living for?

What good is being super healthy, eating nutrient dense foods, and then dying alone with no connections or love to show for our lives? What exactly do we want to be healthy for?

Take some time to evaluate the relationships you currently have, the ones you want to cultivate, and even the ones you might consider terminating for the sake of your emotional and mental health.

Consider reconciling with an estranged family member, making a new friend at work, planning a quiet evening with your significant other, or taking your children on a short day trip to somewhere memorable. If you are lacking relationships and love in your life, don't just sit at home.

Get involved with a community group, a local church, or a Meetup group. If you don't have them already, you can find people who will be meaningful companions in your life. If you need further motivation to do so, just remember – your health depends on it.

Work

We spend about a third of our lives at work. Take out the sleeping part, and most of our adult lives are actually spent working. We are meant to work. We are designed to get things done, to realize accomplishments, to – as George Bernard Shaw put it – "have it make a difference that we lived at all." Work gives meaning to our lives, and without meaning, we humans are lost.

The problem is, too much of our work in the modern world ignores the physical labor part. (We'll get to that in the next section.) And so the majority of us spend our workdays sitting with poor posture at our desks, glued to computer screens or telephones, lacking exposure to sunlight and fresh air.

And all too often, the work we do has no connection to a sense of purpose - which, as humans, we all have and need to see realized in the work we do. If we're going to spend the majority of our waking hours working, we want to know that it means something, that it matters, that the work is bearing fruit.

This is why, even though they don't get paid much money, people like farmers and teachers have traditionally reported great satisfaction in what they do. So do people who stay at home to care for families, or those who do volunteer work or ministry. They see the harvest in that fresh basket of tomatoes, in the kid who finally has the light bulb come on, in the difference they've made in the life of someone in need.

Most of us owe our jobs and livelihoods to corporate America in one way or another, though. And so, it often feels hopeless when our job doesn't, on the surface, provide that clear sense of purpose.

Is it worth it, we might reasonably wonder, to report to a job every day that kills our souls? Well, it's critical to earn a living, this much is true. So just quitting a job isn't really a viable option.

But for the purpose of the bigger picture, it's important to do one of two things. We all need to find work that we love, or find a way to love the work we do. This requires going out on a limb and taking a risk to discover what that might be, or how to reorganize the job we have in a way that it more closely aligns with our values.

Are you already happy in your job? Wonderful! If not, consider these three brief tips for making it a better position – or for finding a new one:

1.   **Commit to a positive attitude**. It's infectious, and if you take the time to make every interaction with your coworkers, boss, employees, or clients a meaningful encounter, then you will certainly find meaning in your day. Eventually, you will also brighten the atmosphere in your workplace.

2.   **Find ways in your job to be able to give to other people**. Real happiness comes from doing for others, so give abundantly! Offer to help people with jobs when you can, bring flowers for a coworker's desk, share some of your new healthy recipes during your lunch break. You'd be surprised what a difference this approach can make.

3.   **If this just isn't the right fit for you, start dreaming**. What are your gifts and talents? What is your God-given genius that you are meant to share with the world? Spend some time with these questions, and then consider whether you can find a way to bring these talents into the work you do now, or what profession would make better use of the skills you have to offer.

Movement

Our bodies are meant to move! We don't need to get a physical exam with a detailed medical report to show us how true this is. We just need to take a brisk walk on a cool morning to know that we feel better and are more energized and grounded from giving our body what it needs.

But in our society, we resist this basic physical desire. A big reason why is because we don't properly fuel our bodies with natural, whole foods. When we do, we begin to feel our bodies the way they are meant to be felt, and we are more driven to exercise.

Purposeful movement and physical activity releases endorphins throughout our bodies that enhance our sense of well being. For some of us, this means hours at the gym and intense workouts.

For most of us, a much more simple approach will work. Walking is the most natural thing to do, and exactly what our bodies are made to do. If you are able to fit a half hour walk into your daily routine each day, even at a leisurely pace, it will do wonders for your body, mind, and soul.

But there are as many ways to move as there are people in this world. Perhaps you prefer weight training, jogging, cycling, swimming, yoga, pilates, Zumba, rebounding, tennis, basketball, skiing, gymnastics – you can do anything!

The key is to find the physical activities you truly enjoy. Your preferences may change with the seasons – and with the seasons of your life. Maybe you ski in winter and swim in summer, and stick with the walking and biking for when the weather is more temperate. Maybe team sports are your thing in your 20's, but something more solitary and peaceful appeals to you in your 60's.

As in food, you need to take the time to experiment and come up with a routine that not only works for you, but that you want to participate in. If it requires will power or struggle, it's not natural for you, and it won't last.

Physical activity also refers to sleep, another essential component of our overall health. Getting just the right amount for you is best achieved when you set the stage for a good night's sleep - turn off the computer and television at least an hour before bed, decompress with a good book and some tea or some meditation and a hot shower, and try to clear your mind.

Hopefully you'll have gotten some movement in during the day, which always helps you sleep better at night.

Making lasting changes is what matters. If you overwhelm yourself at the beginning, you'll be setting yourself up for failure.

While these four areas – spirituality, relationships, work and movement – are critically important to our holistic health, a diet of real, nutritious whole foods is what fuels all of those areas. Eat well, and your connection with the universe will be clearer, your relationships will bloom, you'll be more focused in your work, and your workouts will be much more effective.

Food changes everything!

Chapter 5

The Importance of Support and Community

You want to know what made Weight Watchers and Jenny Craig such popular weight loss programs? It wasn't the packaged foods or the point system.

It was the support.

It was the fact that people who wanted to lose weight didn't feel so isolated. They felt – and continue to feel – like they have a group of people who can empathize with their struggles and give them encouragement when they feel like they can't hang on.

No one has ever achieved optimum health all alone. Part of the reason is that isolation itself is an unhealthy habit... again, if taken to excess.

We are a social species, and we need others around us... not just for social reasons, work reasons, and family reasons. We need others around us for support, community, guidance, and accountability.

We live in a society where potential sabotage lurks around every corner. It lurks in the form of processed foods designed to steal from our taste buds the joy of eating real foods. It lurks in the confusing and untrue health claims made on the outside of packaged foods.

It lurks in the form of sedentary jobs, followed by evenings spent in front of the television and other mindless forms of entertainment that keep us from getting up and moving to entertain ourselves.

And it lurks in social gatherings, restaurants, and the media.

Not only does losing weight and getting healthy seem like too much work, but also it's overwhelming just thinking about where to begin, and how to sustain the effort.

Support in the form of a group of people who have the same goals can be very valuable. But personal, one-on-one support and guidance from a trained professional can also be just what you need.

Imagine having someone with specialized knowledge and the ability to apply it directly to you, dedicated to personally helping you wade through all the unique factors that conspire to keep you unhealthy!

Because everyone is different, a professional is trained to ask the right questions from a more objective place when experimenting with what changes will and won't work for you. They will have a lot of information and knowledge to share, but the most important thing they will offer is support in helping you navigate through all the overwhelming and confusing information to uncover the truth about what uniquely works for you. You will not only receive an array of tools, articles and customized recommendations, but you will also be empowered to thrive in your new, healthy way of life forever.

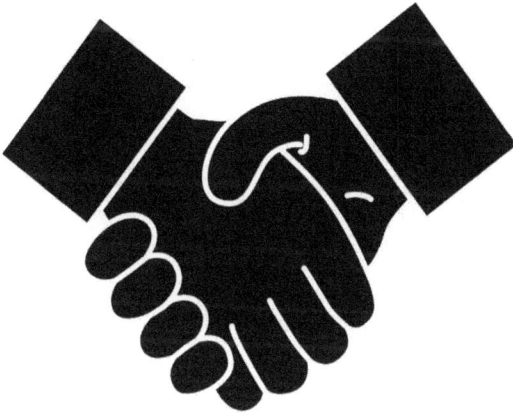

Key #5

Get A Buddy!

If, like many people, you find going it alone to be too difficult, there are people and places you can turn to for support. Enlist a friend, join a Meetup group or get help from a professional!

This will help you gain clarity about your current situation from the very start. You'll begin to understand the factors that are getting in your way, and you'll see the path to health and wellness beyond what you imagined.

Move Past Obstacles

It can also be helpful to break down and address the three primary obstacles to making lasting changes:

**1.	I don't want to give up my favorite foods.**

You don't have to give up your favorite foods! But you can begin to add some new favorite foods to your diet. With a little trial and error, you will figure out the healthy foods you love. You can focus more on "crowding out" the less healthy options rather than "giving up" those options altogether. In other words, the more healthy foods and behaviors you begin to incorporate, the less room you'll have for the less healthy ones. But the focus is on adding positives, not eliminating negatives.

2.   It's too hard to make all these changes at once.

It IS hard to make too many changes at once. And for most people, such attempts fail. That's why we don't make all the changes at once. The body is very resilient and responds well to even the smallest changes intended to yield improvements. Improvements you'll feel empowered to maintain and improve upon - for the rest of your life. Remember, it's not a race to "get there" as fast as you can. The point is to make lasting changes that will add years to your life and life to your years.

3.   It's too confusing to know exactly what to do.

The confusion in the world of food and nutrition these days is crazy. Take time to learn about how to benefit from nutrient density, healthy cooking techniques, what food labels and ingredients really mean, how and where to shop. Custom tailor a plan that works for your body and in your life. Because remember, one size DOES NOT fit all. A book or a program can get you started in the right direction. But it takes time, patience, and support to get where you ultimately need to go.

Take Action !
The 5 Keys to Kickstart
Your Health

Key #1 – Awareness
Use a journal or smartphone app to track what you eat and how you feel. Awareness is the first step toward healthy living.

Key #2 - Upgrade Your Foods
Get lots of greens, lots of vegetables and plenty of water.

Key #3 - Prepare For Success
Plan ahead. Pack and keep these handy at work and on the road: nuts, veggies, fruit and whole food bars.

Key #4 - Balance Your Circle of Life
Fill yourself up with healthy relationships, thoughtful spirituality, meaningful work and energizing physical activity.

Key #5 - Get A Buddy
No one has ever achieved optimum health alone. We need each other for support, guidance, community and accountability.

Encouragement

The best action you can take is to set an example by maximizing your own health. When you upgrade your life, your family and friends will see the changes. They may not say anything immediately nor will they adopt any changes for quite some time. Rest assured, though, they are on notice. Soon, they will see improvements in your health and energy. Then, they will want the same for themselves!

I hope this book has helped you make some simple but significant changes in your health already. There isn't a one size fits all solution to our health, but it's an ironic truth that replacing technology, efficiency and convenience with nourishment, authenticity, and joy yields the most amazing results.

It's by simplifying, not complicating, our approach to life that we can lead a richer and fuller one.

I wish you all the best!

About The Author

Marie Ann Mosher is an Academy of Sports Medicine Certified Personal Trainer and Internationally Certified Integrative Health Coach. She is graduate of the University of Connecticut, where she studied Nutritional Science as well as Occupational Health and Safety. Marie is also a graduate of the Institute for Integrative Nutrition in New York City, where she studied more than one hundred dietary theories and a variety of practical lifestyle teaching methods with some of the world's top health and wellness experts. She's written many books including Beyond Food, The Secret Ingredient, Secret Weight Loss Hacks and the Biohacker Secrets Series.

Marie also hosts the Secret Weight Loss Hacks Free Facebook support community. You can join here - https://www.facebook.com/groups/secretweightlosshacks/

Please visit **www.marieannmosher.com** for more support and free recipes.

Invite Marie to Speak to Your Group or Organization

Marie is an inspiring and dynamic professional speaker. Her audiences include groups and organizations of every size and type.

Topic Specialties:

Individualized Optimal Nutrition
Healing through Primary Food
Self Care Mastery
Stress Management
Lifestyle Balance

For more information go to
www.marieannmosher.com

Connect with Marie

www.marieannmosher.com

www.facebook.com/marieannseaton

www.twitter.com/marieannseaton

www.linkedin.com/in/marieannseaton

www.instagram.com/marieannseaton